BREATHE!

THE
BREATHE!
JOURNAL

**Quit Smoking in 6 weeks using
The Quit Smoking Formula**

QuitSmokingFormula.Com

NAME: _____________________________________

PICK A QUIT DATE WITHIN 14 DAYS FROM TODAY!

I will quit smoking cigarettes on –

DAY _____________________________________

MONTH _________________________________

YEAR __________________________________

TIME __________________________________

LOCATION _____________________________

QuitSmokingFormula.Com

Congratulations on your resolve to quit smoking!

What are the 3 main reasons you want to quit smoking?

1.____

____

2.____

____

3.____

____

Every attempt to quit improves the chance of eventual success. Let's make this your last!

It is time ....

-To breathe better
-To feel better
-To smell better
-To taste better
-To be healthier
-To experience more energy
-To save money
-To protect your loved ones from secondhand smoke

The BREATHE! Journal was made to help you quit smoking. It is best used with The Quit Smoking Formula (QSF), an online course designed to help you quit smoking in 6 weeks.

The Quit Smoking Formula (QSF) is a proven strategy that utilizes the principles of Cognitive-Behavioural Therapy, Directed Action, Mindset Shift, Medication-Assisted Treatment, Lifestyle Changes, and a proven roadmap to help you quit smoking.

The Quit Smoking Formula is made up of 5 steps that make up the acronym SMILE

S - Starting your smoke-free life

M - Mastering your mind

I - Improving your chances to Quit once and for all

L - Lifestyle Changes to heal your body.

E - Ensuring long term success

QuitSmokingFormula.Com

Identifying Your Smoking Triggers

✔ Check Your Key Triggers

- ☐ Nicotine cravings
- ☐ When I have a task to do
- ☐ When I wake up
- ☐ After eating
- ☐ When I need an energy boost
- ☐ To concentrate better
- ☐ When I need to relax
- ☐ When I'm bored
- ☐ When I'm stressed at work

.....there's more!

Identifying Your Smoking Triggers

✓ Check Your Key Triggers

- ☐ While driving
- ☐ When I'm taking a break at work
- ☐ When I feel down or depressed
- ☐ When I'm angry
- ☐ When I feel great
- ☐ Talking on the telephone
- ☐ Social situations
- ☐ After coffee
- ☐ When I drink alcohol
- ☐ Others _______________________________________

____

____

Getting Support

- Tell family and friends you are quitting and inform them of your quit date
- Ask your partner or a friend to quit with you
- Request people living with you smoke outside
- Call a quit line for support
- Consider joining a FaceBook support group
- Make a list of 3 people who can support you

Write down the names of 3 people you can call for support

1.______________________________________

2.______________________________________

3.______________________________________

**Join Our FaceBook Group
"Quit Smoking SUCCESS Group"**

Getting Ready to Quit

Making small behavioral changes will help break up your smoking routine and severe the link between your triggers and smoking.

Check one or more of the suggestions below and try to stick with them. Only add some more as you get used to the ones you picked.

- [ ] Try switching to a brand of cigarettes you don't like
- [ ] Hold your cigarettes in your opposite hand
- [ ] Only buy one pack at a time
- [ ] Avoid your favorite smoking places eg car, patio
- [ ] Stop carrying cigarettes on you
- [ ] Each time you want a cigarette, wait 5 minutes
- [ ] Delay each cigarette with other activities such as taking a walk, chewing on sugar-free gum
- [ ] Delay your first cigarette of the day by 1 hour
- [ ] Eat a fruit after meals, rather than smoke
- [ ] Decrease the places and situations to smoke
- [ ] Only smoke if you absolutely need to. Not out of habit

.....there's more!

Getting Ready to Quit

Making small behavioral changes will help break up your smoking routine and severe the link between your triggers and smoking.

Check one or more of the suggestions below and try to stick with them. Only add some more as you get used to the ones you picked.

- [ ] Do not smoke indoors
- [ ] Discard your cigarette after smoking half of it
- [ ] Smoke only during even or odd hours of the day
- [ ] Give up 1-3 cigarettes you can do without daily
- [ ] Avoid emptying your ashtray as a reminder
- [ ] If you can, look in a mirror each time you light up
- [ ] Change your "smoke breaks" to "walk breaks"
- [ ] Ask others not to smoke around you
- [ ] Avoid smoking areas such as bars
- [ ] Keep your hands busy
- [ ] Engage in a hobby to help distract you
- [ ] Consider smoking cessation medications
- [ ] Pick a quit day that is as stress-free as possible
- [ ] Take it one day at a time. Do not overthink it

Strategies To Use After You Quit

- Spend time in places where smoking is not allowed
- Avoid situations you associate with smoking
- Cut down on caffeine and sugar. Drink lots of water
- Avoid alcohol and coffee if these make you smoke
- Keep your hands busy with a coin, paper clip, or pen
- Occupy your mouth with cinnamon sticks, toothpicks, carrots, celery, or sugarless gum
- Give yourself a treat and plan for future treats
- Detail your car, wash your clothes, clean your house
- Brush your teeth more often
- Use mouthwash regularly
- Go for walks, exercise regularly
- Consider staying away from your smoking social groups, at least initially
- Make sure you get good sleep. 7-8 hrs daily is ideal
- Keep yourself busy with a new hobby
- Find coping mechanisms to manage your stress
- Consider treating ongoing mental health conditions
- Continue smoking cessation medications per prescription
- Never consider "just one cigarette"
- Join a support group for motivation to keep going
- Enjoy life as a non-smoker

"The best time to quit smoking was the day you started, the second best time to quit is today." – Anonymous

QUIT.

BREATHE.

LIVE.

Day Number:__________   Date:______________

Did you smoke today? ______________

If No, well done!!!   If Yes, how many? ________

Describe your withdrawals and cravings

____

____

____

What coping mechanisms have you found helpful

____

____

What do you plan to do differently?

____

____

How is your mood? ________________________________

How much money did you save today?____________

What did you do today to help heal your body
(eating better, taking supplements, sleeping better,
exercising) ____________________________________

"Energy and persistence conquer all things." –
Benjamin Franklin

Journal your thoughts ....

Day Number:________   Date:____________

Did you smoke today? ____________

If No, well done!!!   ●   If Yes, how many? ______

Describe your withdrawals and cravings

____

____

____

What coping mechanisms have you found helpful

____

____

What do you plan to do differently?

____

____

How is your mood? ______________________________

How much money did you save today?____________

What did you do today to help heal your body
(eating better, taking supplements, sleeping better,
exercising) ______________________________________

"Only I can change my life. No one can do it for me." - Carol Burnett

Journal your thoughts ....

Day Number:_________   Date:_____________

Did you smoke today? ______________

If No, well done!!!   •   If Yes, how many? _______

Describe your withdrawals and cravings

____

____

____

What coping mechanisms have you found helpful

____

____

What do you plan to do differently?

____

____

How is your mood? ____________________________

How much money did you save today?___________

What did you do today to help heal your body
(eating better, taking supplements, sleeping better,
exercising) ____________________________________

"Strength does not come from winning. Your struggles develop your strengths. When you go through hardships and decide not to surrender, that is strength." - Arnold Schwarzenegger

Journal your thoughts ....

Day Number:__________   Date:____________

Did you smoke today? ____________

If No, well done!!!   ●   If Yes, how many? ______

Describe your withdrawals and cravings

____

____

____

What coping mechanisms have you found helpful

____

____

What do you plan to do differently?

____

____

How is your mood? ______________________________

How much money did you save today?____________

What did you do today to help heal your body
(eating better, taking supplements, sleeping better,
exercising) ______________________________________

"The will to win, the desire to succeed, the urge to reach your full potential ...these are the keys that will unlock the door to personal excellence." - Confucius

Journal your thoughts ....

Day Number:__________   Date:______________

Did you smoke today? ______________

If No, well done!!!   ●   If Yes, how many? ________

Describe your withdrawals and cravings

____

____

____

What coping mechanisms have you found helpful

____

____

What do you plan to do differently?

____

____

How is your mood? ____________________

How much money did you save today?__________

What did you do today to help heal your body
(eating better, taking supplements, sleeping better,
exercising) ____________________________

"Our greatest weakness lies in giving up. The most certain way to succeed is always to try just one more time." – Thomas Edison

Journal your thoughts ....

Day Number:___________   Date:_______________

Did you smoke today? _____________

If No, well done!!!   ●   If Yes, how many? _______

Describe your withdrawals and cravings

____

____

____

What coping mechanisms have you found helpful

____

____

What do you plan to do differently?

____

____

How is your mood? ______________________________

How much money did you save today?_____________

What did you do today to help heal your body
(eating better, taking supplements, sleeping better,
exercising) _____________________________________

"It always seems impossible until it's done." –
Nelson Mandela

Journal your thoughts ....

Day Number:_________   Date:____________

Did you smoke today? ______________

If No, well done!!!   If Yes, how many? _______

Describe your withdrawals and cravings

____

____

____

What coping mechanisms have you found helpful

____

____

What do you plan to do differently?

____

____

How is your mood? ______________________________

How much money did you save today?____________

What did you do today to help heal your body
(eating better, taking supplements, sleeping better,
exercising) _____________________________________

"Our greatest glory is not in never failing but in rising up every time we fail." - Ralph Waldo Emerson

Journal your thoughts ....

Day Number:_________   Date:____________

Did you smoke today? ____________

If No, well done!!!   If Yes, how many? _______

Describe your withdrawals and cravings

____

____

____

What coping mechanisms have you found helpful

____

____

What do you plan to do differently?

____

____

How is your mood? ______________________________

How much money did you save today?____________

What did you do today to help heal your body
(eating better, taking supplements, sleeping better,
exercising) _____________________________________

"People often say that motivation doesn't last. Well, neither does bathing – that's why we recommend it daily." – Zig Ziglar

Journal your thoughts ....

Day Number:___________   Date:______________

Did you smoke today? ______________

If No, well done!!! ● If Yes, how many? ________

Describe your withdrawals and cravings

____

____

____

What coping mechanisms have you found helpful

____

____

What do you plan to do differently?

____

____

How is your mood? _____________________________

How much money did you save today?____________

What did you do today to help heal your body
(eating better, taking supplements, sleeping better,
exercising) _____________________________________

"When you are going through hell, keep on going.
Never never never give up." - Winston Churchill

Journal your thoughts ....

Day Number:________   Date:___________

Did you smoke today? ____________

If No, well done!!!   ●   If Yes, how many? ______

Describe your withdrawals and cravings

____

____

____

What coping mechanisms have you found helpful

____

____

What do you plan to do differently?

____

____

How is your mood? ______________________________

How much money did you save today?___________

What did you do today to help heal your body (eating better, taking supplements, sleeping better, exercising) _______________________________

"Don't let the fear of the time it will take to accomplish something stand in the way of your doing it. The time will pass anyway; we might as well put that passing time to the best possible use." – Earl Nightingale

Journal your thoughts ....

Day Number:__________   Date:______________

Did you smoke today? ______________

If No, well done!!!   ●   If Yes, how many? ________

Describe your withdrawals and cravings

____

____

____

What coping mechanisms have you found helpful

____

____

What do you plan to do differently?

____

____

How is your mood? ______________________________

How much money did you save today?____________

What did you do today to help heal your body
(eating better, taking supplements, sleeping better,
exercising) _____________________________________

"It does not matter how slowly you go so long as you do not stop." - Confucius

Journal your thoughts ....

Day Number:__________   Date:____________

Did you smoke today? ______________

If No, well done!!!   ●   If Yes, how many? ________

Describe your withdrawals and cravings

____

____

____

What coping mechanisms have you found helpful

____

____

What do you plan to do differently?

____

____

How is your mood? _______________________________

How much money did you save today?____________

What did you do today to help heal your body
(eating better, taking supplements, sleeping better,
exercising) ______________________________________

"I am not discouraged because every wrong attempt discarded is a step forward." - Thomas Edison

Journal your thoughts ....

Day Number:________   Date:___________

Did you smoke today? ____________

If No, well done!!!   If Yes, how many? ______

Describe your withdrawals and cravings

____

____

____

What coping mechanisms have you found helpful

____

____

What do you plan to do differently?

____

____

How is your mood? ______________________________

How much money did you save today?____________

What did you do today to help heal your body
(eating better, taking supplements, sleeping better,
exercising) ______________________________________

"It's not that I'm so smart, it's just that I stay with problems longer." - Albert Einstein

Journal your thoughts ....

Day Number:________   Date:___________

Did you smoke today? ____________

If No, well done!!!   ●   If Yes, how many? _______

Describe your withdrawals and cravings

____

____

____

What coping mechanisms have you found helpful

____

____

What do you plan to do differently?

____

____

How is your mood? _______________________________

How much money did you save today?___________

What did you do today to help heal your body
(eating better, taking supplements, sleeping better,
exercising) ______________________________________

"Success is the sum of small efforts, repeated day in and day out." - Robert Collier

Journal your thoughts ....

Day Number:__________   Date:____________

Did you smoke today? ____________

If No, well done!!!   ⬤   If Yes, how many? ______

Describe your withdrawals and cravings

____

____

____

What coping mechanisms have you found helpful

____

____

What do you plan to do differently?

____

____

How is your mood? _____________________________

How much money did you save today?____________

What did you do today to help heal your body
(eating better, taking supplements, sleeping better,
exercising) _____________________________________

"Cigarettes are killers that travel in packs." – Anonymous

Journal your thoughts ....

Day Number:_______   Date:__________

Did you smoke today? ___________

If No, well done!!! ● If Yes, how many? ______

Describe your withdrawals and cravings

____

____

____

What coping mechanisms have you found helpful

____

____

What do you plan to do differently?

____

____

How is your mood? _________________________

How much money did you save today?__________

What did you do today to help heal your body
(eating better, taking supplements, sleeping better,
exercising) _______________________________

"Our strength grows out of our weakness." - Ralph
Waldo Emerson

Journal your thoughts ....

Day Number:_________   Date:____________

Did you smoke today? _____________

If No, well done!!!   ●   If Yes, how many? _______

Describe your withdrawals and cravings

____

____

____

What coping mechanisms have you found helpful

____

____

What do you plan to do differently?

____

____

How is your mood? _______________________________

How much money did you save today?____________

What did you do today to help heal your body
(eating better, taking supplements, sleeping better,
exercising) _____________________________________

"At least three times every day take a moment and ask yourself what is really important. Have the wisdom and the courage to build your life around your answer." - Lee Jampolsky

Journal your thoughts ....

Day Number:__________   Date:______________

Did you smoke today? ______________

If No, well done!!!   ●   If Yes, how many? ________

Describe your withdrawals and cravings

____

____

____

What coping mechanisms have you found helpful

____

____

What do you plan to do differently?

____

____

How is your mood? ______________________________

How much money did you save today?____________

What did you do today to help heal your body
(eating better, taking supplements, sleeping better,
exercising) ________________________________

"Your craving is temporary but the damage to your lungs is permanent." - Anonymous

Journal your thoughts ....

Day Number:___________   Date:_______________

Did you smoke today? _______________

If No, well done!!!   ●   If Yes, how many? _______

Describe your withdrawals and cravings

____

____

____

What coping mechanisms have you found helpful

____

____

What do you plan to do differently?

____

____

How is your mood? ______________________________

How much money did you save today?_____________

What did you do today to help heal your body
(eating better, taking supplements, sleeping better,
exercising) ______________________________________

"Checking your ego, abandoning it, letting go, is a huge part of recovery from addiction." - Susannah Grant

Journal your thoughts ....

Day Number:_________   Date:____________

Did you smoke today? ____________

If No, well done!!!   If Yes, how many? ______

Describe your withdrawals and cravings

____

____

____

What coping mechanisms have you found helpful

____

____

What do you plan to do differently?

____

____

How is your mood? __________________________

How much money did you save today?__________

What did you do today to help heal your body
(eating better, taking supplements, sleeping better,
exercising) _________________________________

"Gift your lungs oxygen not tar. Gift your body exercise not bad health. Gift your lips kisses not cigarette butts. Give yourself a life not death." - Anonymous

Journal your thoughts ....

Day Number:________   Date:___________

Did you smoke today? ___________

If No, well done!!! ⬤ If Yes, how many? ______

Describe your withdrawals and cravings

____

____

____

What coping mechanisms have you found helpful

____

____

What do you plan to do differently?

____

____

How is your mood? ________________________________

How much money did you save today?_________

What did you do today to help heal your body
(eating better, taking supplements, sleeping better,
exercising) ____________________________________

"Replacing the smoke on your face with a smile today will replace illness in your life with happiness tomorrow." - Anonymous

Journal your thoughts ....

Day Number:_________   Date:____________

Did you smoke today? ____________

If No, well done!!!   ●   If Yes, how many? _______

Describe your withdrawals and cravings

____

____

____

What coping mechanisms have you found helpful

____

____

What do you plan to do differently?

____

____

How is your mood? ______________________________

How much money did you save today?____________

What did you do today to help heal your body
(eating better, taking supplements, sleeping better,
exercising) ______________________________________

"There is no such thing in anyone's life as an unimportant day." - Alexander Woollcott

Journal your thoughts ....

Day Number:_________   Date:____________

Did you smoke today? ____________

If No, well done!!!   If Yes, how many? _______

Describe your withdrawals and cravings

____

____

____

What coping mechanisms have you found helpful

____

____

What do you plan to do differently?

____

____

How is your mood? ________________________

How much money did you save today?__________

What did you do today to help heal your body
(eating better, taking supplements, sleeping better,
exercising) ______________________________

"Smokers don't grow old .....they die young." – Anonymous

Journal your thoughts ....

Day Number:________   Date:___________

Did you smoke today? ____________

If No, well done!!!   ●   If Yes, how many? ______

Describe your withdrawals and cravings

____

____

____

What coping mechanisms have you found helpful

____

____

What do you plan to do differently?

____

____

How is your mood? ______________________________

How much money did you save today?____________

What did you do today to help heal your body
(eating better, taking supplements, sleeping better,
exercising) _____________________________________

"A cigarette says: Today you turn me into ashes, but tomorrow is my turn." - Anonymous

Journal your thoughts ....

Day Number:_______ Date:__________

Did you smoke today? ____________

If No, well done!!! ● If Yes, how many? ______

Describe your withdrawals and cravings

____
____
____

What coping mechanisms have you found helpful

____
____

What do you plan to do differently?

____
____

How is your mood? ______________________

How much money did you save today?__________

What did you do today to help heal your body (eating better, taking supplements, sleeping better, exercising) ________________________

"We are what we repeatedly do. Excellence, then, is not an act, but a habit." – Aristotle

Journal your thoughts ....

Day Number:__________   Date:____________

Did you smoke today? ____________

If No, well done!!!   ●   If Yes, how many? ______

Describe your withdrawals and cravings

____

____

____

What coping mechanisms have you found helpful

____

____

What do you plan to do differently?

____

____

How is your mood? _____________________________

How much money did you save today?___________

What did you do today to help heal your body
(eating better, taking supplements, sleeping better,
exercising) _____________________________________

"Your life is in your hands, to make of it what you chose." - Anonymous

Journal your thoughts ....

Day Number:_________   Date:___________

Did you smoke today? _____________

If No, well done!!!   ●   If Yes, how many? _______

Describe your withdrawals and cravings

____

____

____

What coping mechanisms have you found helpful

____

____

What do you plan to do differently?

____

____

How is your mood? _______________________________

How much money did you save today?___________

What did you do today to help heal your body
(eating better, taking supplements, sleeping better,
exercising) ______________________________________

"Health is not everything, but without health, everything else is nothing." – Anonymous

Journal your thoughts ....

Day Number:_________   Date:____________

Did you smoke today? _____________

If No, well done!!!   If Yes, how many? _______

Describe your withdrawals and cravings

____

____

____

What coping mechanisms have you found helpful

____

____

What do you plan to do differently?

____

____

How is your mood? ______________________________

How much money did you save today?__________

What did you do today to help heal your body
(eating better, taking supplements, sleeping better,
exercising) _____________________________

"Smoking is a habit that drains your money and kills you slowly, one puff after another. Quit smoking, start living." – Anonymous

Journal your thoughts ....

Day Number:_______   Date:___________

Did you smoke today? ___________

If No, well done!!! ● If Yes, how many? ______

Describe your withdrawals and cravings

____

____

____

What coping mechanisms have you found helpful

____

____

What do you plan to do differently?

____

____

How is your mood? _____________________

How much money did you save today?_________

What did you do today to help heal your body (eating better, taking supplements, sleeping better, exercising) ____________________________

"A cigarette is the only consumer product which when used as directed kills its consumer." – Anonymous

Journal your thoughts ....

Day Number:_________   Date:____________

Did you smoke today? ____________

If No, well done!!! ● If Yes, how many? _______

Describe your withdrawals and cravings

____

____

____

What coping mechanisms have you found helpful

____

____

What do you plan to do differently?

____

____

How is your mood? ______________________________

How much money did you save today?___________

What did you do today to help heal your body
(eating better, taking supplements, sleeping better,
exercising) _______________________________________

"It is in your moments of decision that your destiny is shaped." – Tony Robbins

Journal your thoughts ....

Day Number:_________   Date:______________

Did you smoke today? _____________

If No, well done!!!   ●   If Yes, how many? _______

Describe your withdrawals and cravings

____

____

____

What coping mechanisms have you found helpful

____

____

What do you plan to do differently?

____

____

How is your mood? _______________________________

How much money did you save today?____________

What did you do today to help heal your body
(eating better, taking supplements, sleeping better,
exercising) _______________________________________

"Smoking cigarettes is like paying to have your life cut shorter." – Anonymous

Journal your thoughts ....

Day Number:___________   Date:_______________

Did you smoke today? _______________

If No, well done!!!   ●   If Yes, how many? _______

Describe your withdrawals and cravings

____

____

____

What coping mechanisms have you found helpful

____

____

What do you plan to do differently?

____

____

How is your mood? _______________________________

How much money did you save today?_____________

What did you do today to help heal your body
(eating better, taking supplements, sleeping better,
exercising) _______________________________________

"Burn calories, not cigarettes." – Anonymous

Journal your thoughts ....

Day Number:__________   Date:____________

Did you smoke today? ____________

If No, well done!!!   ⬤   If Yes, how many? ______

Describe your withdrawals and cravings

____

____

____

What coping mechanisms have you found helpful

____

____

What do you plan to do differently?

____

____

How is your mood? ______________________________

How much money did you save today?____________

What did you do today to help heal your body
(eating better, taking supplements, sleeping better,
exercising) ______________________________________

"Tar the roads, not your lungs." – Anonymous

Journal your thoughts ....

Day Number:________   Date:___________

Did you smoke today? ____________

If No, well done!!!   ●   If Yes, how many? ______

Describe your withdrawals and cravings

____

____

____

What coping mechanisms have you found helpful

____

____

What do you plan to do differently?

____

____

How is your mood? _____________________________

How much money did you save today?___________

What did you do today to help heal your body
(eating better, taking supplements, sleeping better,
exercising) ___________________________________

"What lies in our power to do, lies in our power not to do." – Aristotle

Journal your thoughts ....

Day Number:__________   Date:____________

Did you smoke today? ____________

If No, well done!!!   ⬤   If Yes, how many? ______

Describe your withdrawals and cravings

____

____

____

What coping mechanisms have you found helpful

____

____

What do you plan to do differently?

____

____

How is your mood? _____________________________

How much money did you save today?___________

What did you do today to help heal your body
(eating better, taking supplements, sleeping better,
exercising) _____________________________________

"Life's vibrant hues are way too beautiful and precious to be distorted by the smoke of cigarettes."
– Anonymous

Journal your thoughts ....

Day Number:____________   Date:______________

Did you smoke today? ______________

If No, well done!!!   If Yes, how many? ________

Describe your withdrawals and cravings

____

____

____

What coping mechanisms have you found helpful

____

____

What do you plan to do differently?

____

____

How is your mood? _______________________________

How much money did you save today?____________

What did you do today to help heal your body
(eating better, taking supplements, sleeping better,
exercising) _____________________________________

"A cigarette a day keeps the doctor in pay." –
Anonymous

Journal your thoughts ....

Day Number:________   Date:___________

Did you smoke today? ____________

If No, well done!!!   If Yes, how many? ______

Describe your withdrawals and cravings

____

____

____

What coping mechanisms have you found helpful

____

____

What do you plan to do differently?

____

____

How is your mood? _____________________________

How much money did you save today?___________

What did you do today to help heal your body
(eating better, taking supplements, sleeping better,
exercising) _____________________________________

"Disadvantages of smoking are many but those of quitting are none. Advantages of smoking are none but those of quitting are many." – Anonymous

Journal your thoughts ....

Day Number:__________   Date:______________

Did you smoke today? ______________

If No, well done!!!   ●   If Yes, how many? ________

Describe your withdrawals and cravings

____

____

____

What coping mechanisms have you found helpful

____

____

What do you plan to do differently?

____

____

How is your mood? ________________________________

How much money did you save today?___________

What did you do today to help heal your body
(eating better, taking supplements, sleeping better,
exercising) ______________________________________

"The secret of getting ahead is getting started." – Mark Twain

Journal your thoughts ....

Day Number:_________   Date:___________

Did you smoke today? ____________

If No, well done!!! ● If Yes, how many? ______

Describe your withdrawals and cravings

____

____

____

What coping mechanisms have you found helpful

____

____

What do you plan to do differently?

____

____

How is your mood? _____________________

How much money did you save today?_________

What did you do today to help heal your body
(eating better, taking supplements, sleeping better,
exercising) _______________________________

"The surest way not to fail is to determine to succeed." – Richard Brinsley Sheridan

Journal your thoughts ....

Day Number:_________   Date:___________

Did you smoke today? ____________

If No, well done!!!   ●   If Yes, how many? ______

Describe your withdrawals and cravings

____

____

____

What coping mechanisms have you found helpful

____

____

What do you plan to do differently?

____

____

How is your mood? ______________________________

How much money did you save today?___________

What did you do today to help heal your body
(eating better, taking supplements, sleeping better,
exercising) _____________________________________

"Believe you can and you're halfway there." – Theodore Roosevelt

Journal your thoughts ....

Day Number:__________   Date:____________

Did you smoke today? ____________

If No, well done!!!   ●   If Yes, how many? ______

Describe your withdrawals and cravings
____

____

____

What coping mechanisms have you found helpful
____

____

What do you plan to do differently?
____

____

How is your mood? ____________________

How much money did you save today?__________

What did you do today to help heal your body
(eating better, taking supplements, sleeping better,
exercising) ___________________________

"Good habits are just as addictive as bad habits. But much more rewarding." – Anonymous

Journal your thoughts ....

Day Number:_________   Date:___________

Did you smoke today? ____________

If No, well done!!!   ⬤   If Yes, how many? _______

Describe your withdrawals and cravings

____

____

____

What coping mechanisms have you found helpful

____

____

What do you plan to do differently?

____

____

How is your mood? ______________________________

How much money did you save today?___________

What did you do today to help heal your body
(eating better, taking supplements, sleeping better,
exercising) ______________________________________

"The man who moves a mountain begins by carrying away small stones." – Confucius

Journal your thoughts ....

Day Number:________   Date:____________

Did you smoke today? ____________

If No, well done!!!   ⬤   If Yes, how many? ______

Describe your withdrawals and cravings

____

____

____

What coping mechanisms have you found helpful

____

____

What do you plan to do differently?

____

____

How is your mood? _______________________________

How much money did you save today?____________

What did you do today to help heal your body
(eating better, taking supplements, sleeping better,
exercising) _______________________________________

"Don't exchange what you want most for what you want at that moment." – Anonymous

Journal your thoughts ....

Day Number:________   Date:___________

Did you smoke today? ____________

If No, well done!!! ● If Yes, how many? _______

Describe your withdrawals and cravings

____

____

____

What coping mechanisms have you found helpful

____

____

What do you plan to do differently?

____

____

How is your mood? ___________________________

How much money did you save today?___________

What did you do today to help heal your body
(eating better, taking supplements, sleeping better,
exercising) ________________________________

"I count him braver who overcomes his desires than him who conquers his enemies; for the hardest victory is over self." – Aristotle

Journal your thoughts ....

CONGRATULATIONS!

You've been on quite the journey, and you stuck with it! You should be incredibly proud of yourself.

Despite the odds and challenges, you were able to break free from nicotine addiction.

You should see this as a new phase of your life. Begin to enjoy your life as a happy non-smoker!

QUIT. BREATHE. LIVE.

Dr. Air

QuitSmokingFormula.Com

Journal your thoughts ....

QuitSmokingFormula.Com

Journal your thoughts ....

QuitSmokingFormula.Com

Journal your thoughts ....

QuitSmokingFormula.Com

Journal your thoughts ....

QuitSmokingFormula.Com

Journal your thoughts ....

QuitSmokingFormula.Com

Journal your thoughts ....

QuitSmokingFormula.Com

Journal your thoughts ....

QuitSmokingFormula.Com

Journal your thoughts ....

QuitSmokingFormula.Com

Journal your thoughts ....

QuitSmokingFormula.Com

Journal your thoughts ....

QUIT.

BREATHE.

LIVE.

QuitSmokingFormula.Com

www.ingramcontent.com/pod-product-compliance
Lightning Source LLC
Chambersburg PA
CBHW070718250726
48662CB00001B/483